Table of Contents

Understanding the Relationship Between Pelvic and Lower Back Pain

1. Introduction to Pelvic and Lower Back Pain

The relationship between pelvic and low back pain (PLBP) would also be expected to be greater for individuals with possible sources of pelvic pain, such as pregnancy and childbirth, although this remains controversial. Pelvic pain in combination with low back pain usually coincides with an increased psychological burden. The association between pelvic and lower back pain has long been recognized, particularly in the obstetric population. While following childbirth, many women report experiencing pain in the pelvic with concomitant low back, with a prevalence reported at around 20%, with some women continuing to experience pain-related disability for years. In women, PLBP can be acute or chronic. If the onset of PLBP occurs during pregnancy or after childbirth, the pain will usually be classified as pelvic girdle pain. Acute PLBP can be defined as a new episode of unexplained pain, with or without leg pain, that has not been treated successfully within the previous six months.

Pelvic and lower back pain are highly prevalent in the general population and are generally associated with adverse clinical outcomes, including severe disability, impaired quality of life, and substantial hidden healthcare costs. It is difficult to determine if pelvic pain and LBP represent a single condition due to the common possibility of underlying overlapping clinical features. Pelvic pain is commonly described in patients with low back-related leg pain. Such an area in the lower back, such as the sacroiliac joint, can produce pain in the buttock, groin, or leg alone. However, pelvic pain is frequently observed in the population of the general without the presence of lower back or leg pain and is more prevalent in females than in males.

1.1. Definition and Prevalence

Low back pain is one of the most popular conditions in order to reduce workers' productivity from other jobs and it has significant negative effects on companies. Approximately 80 percent of people have had lower back pain at least once in their life, and it is a condition that often recurs. Similarly, striking the worldwide population is very frequent and has consistent poor motor control. However, long-term chronic lower back pain (CLBP) study is scarce in relation to the alignment of the lower extremities and the association between pelvic tilt and low back pain.

Pelvic and low back pain are generally located from the second sacral segment to the L5 and SI regions, affecting the structures of the spine, especially the tissue in the lumbar area. Increased intra-abdominal pressure and low back pain can cause an increase in upper lumbar and vesicular nerve excitability. There has been plenty of discussion among researchers as to how lower back pain, posture, and weak core muscles are related to each other in the literature. Uneven low back pain is clearly a structural and biomechanical issue, whereas pelvic postural distortion is clearly related to disorder in core or postural muscles commonly referred to.

1.2. Impact on Quality of Life

Pelvic organs: uterovesical pouch/posterior fornix/seminal vesicles and rectovesical pouch. Divisum may be a normal anatomical variation in skeletal formations, maintaining the patient's low back as the main complaint and hindering the use of the pelvis (the other in predominantly perineum may have low back pain as the ISG has completed). Also, 29% had a known sacral primary movement disorder such as sacral tilt, separation/rotation, or posterior torsion. It has been shown that sacral torsion can rotate counter-rotating. Joint Disorder – Pubic. To determine the pelvic tilt, inferior landmarks are used in lumbar discography, generally into "low back" or "buttock and/or leg" and/or a combination with "coccyx, buttock, and/or leg pain".

Pelvic girdle pain and low back pain both contribute to decreased quality of life. Other factors may also limit the quality of life in this study group, including previous pregnancy low back pain and/or pelvic girdle pain, and previous sick leave. The impact of low back pain and pelvic girdle pain that are already chronic (i.e., that are ongoing at or beyond 8 weeks postpartum) on an individual mother is important, on the family is important, and when it impacts on primary care and specialist assessment to provide cost-effective treatments. The fact that the impact extends beyond the mother to her partner, baby, family or whanau at home, her workplace whether paid or voluntary, and the allocation of resources is important to maternity and primary care service providers. The impact on society of these pains is in the "domino effects". In other words, a healthy mother experiencing less pain will remain at work, remain in a positive rather than negative relationship, while her healthy partner will work and remain motivated and healthy. This is likely to be a very productive policy when "positive" factors are produced in all the respective parties to the level they each represent for the community well-being.

2. Anatomy of the Pelvic and Lower Back Regions

The Anatomy of the Lower Back Region The lower back, also known as the lumbosacral region, is positioned below the thoracic region of the spine, and below the abdomen. It is made up of five individual vertebrae that start at the bottom of the ribcage, forming what is called the thoracolumbar spine. In between each of these vertebrae are fibrous discs that provide cushioning and protection. An intricate array of ligaments and muscles work together to stabilize the lumbar spine, while providing flexibility and the ability to perform a wide range of movements. The muscles of the lumbar spine represent the 'core' muscles responsible for supporting the body when sitting, walking, running, twisting, bending, and stretching. In addition to bones, the pelvis and lower back are made up of many muscle groups (obturator muscle, iliacus muscle, psoas major muscle, quadratus lumborum, latissimus dorsi muscle, thoracotomy muscle, and rectus abdominis muscle) and joints (that connect the pelvis bone to the vertebral column and the femur bones).

The Anatomy of the Pelvic Region The pelvis is essentially made up of three bones: the pubis, the ischium, and the ilium. Three of the ilium are fused together. The right and left sides of the pelvis are joined together at the rear by the sacrum. Although the surfaces where these three bones meet are bumpy and rough, the bones are held tightly together by several strong ligaments that do not permit much movement between them. The lower parts of the joint surfaces are lined by a thick ring of gristle, called cartilage, upon which weight of the body is supported in an erect position. The joints between the joints of the pelvis form the front of a strong ring. In addition, the surface of the joints is rough and very thick and, to a great extent, reinforced by tough strands of strong fibers. Finally, five large vertebrae (the sacral vertebrae) are cemented together to form a large, wedge-shaped bone situated at the back of the pelvis.

These two sections work together to give readers a detailed look at the composition of the pelvic and lower back regions, with an examination of the structure of bones, muscles, and joints. This will provide the foundational knowledge necessary for readers to make sense of the information presented in the following sections, as these core components are potential sources of pain and discomfort.

2.1. Structures Involved

Nociceptive signaling from the pelvic viscera or local muscles, the anterior or lateral cutaneous nerves, the two major iliac crest and trochanteric bursae, or the sacroiliac joint, which sends nociceptive signals through the dorsal root ganglion not just at the spinal level where it is injured, but also to the afferent nociceptive signal configuration traveling through it. Muscles innervated by the L1, L2, and L3 nerve roots feed nociceptors that send signals to the same second-order neurons or contain its sensory Gerlach's neurons that receive the pelvic nociceptive signals. Thus, upon disinhibition of the phrenic nuclei, pelvic pain sends motor signals that affect the diaphragm and ribcage, resulting in concurrent upper quadrant/ribs/thoracic cage pain or dysfunction. So that both the frontal and dorsal fibers of the psoas major send nociceptive signals to both the lumbar spinal levels and the thoracic/lumbar spinal levels with a summative effect. This is not surprising, as the fibers of the psoas that insert into the spines of T12 and L1 fuse with the deepest fibers of the quadratus lumborum and those attaching from the transverse processes of L1 through 4 to the twelfth rib, both of which send nociceptive signals to thoracic levels. Also, the dual nerve innervation of the psoas major muscle by the L1, 2, and 3 fibers of ventral rami also feed C3, 4 (phrenic) spinal nerve roots. The iliopsoas is innervated by L1, 2, 3 ventral sensory fibers and L2, 3 ventral motor innervation. Posteriorly, the lumbar spine the nociceptive and nocimotor branches of the ventral rami, nerves nervorum, feed local muscles innervated by the same spinal roots as well as the multifidus and erector spinae. The many sinuvertebral nerves send proprioceptive and nociceptive signals that share dorsal horn neurons taking concurrent signals of benign and malignant origin to the spinal cord and thalamus.

First of all, to understand the relationship between pelvic and lower back pain, a brief overview of the structures involved in these dysfunctions is necessary. The pelvis, composed of four bones (the two pelvic bones, the sacrum, and the coccyx), is involved in the attachment of multiple muscle groups and in housing the female reproductive system. It plays a pivotal role in the stabilization of the trunk through its muscular attachments. The lower back, or lumbar spine, is made up of five separate vertebrae, an intervertebral disc between each of them, and multiple joints, ligaments, and muscles that lend to the structure's stability and overall mobility.

2.2. Nerve Pathways

The nervous system that controls the pelvis and lower back can be divided into two main branches. The Peripheral Nervous System (PNS) is going to have influence on the pelvic and lower back areas directly. Yet, there is another set of nerves called the Central Nervous System (CNS). The CNS is basically how things are controlled by the brain and brainstem. It is the central processor that doles out output to all the different areas. Clearly, messing with the CNS operation has potential in how our findings relate to pain locally in the pelvis and back, and also globally, such as IBS and other issues. So, if the nervous system runs through the pelvis and lower back, then it stands to reason that some of our findings could help us understand the mechanics of adherences and how they might influence lower back and pelvic pain.

The nerve pathways associated with the pelvis and lower back are a complex system that actually works across several areas. Many of the nerve pathways actually start in the brain without even touching the pelvis or back, yet still have influence on those areas. The point is, the network of nerves that govern the mechanics of the pelvis and lower back is complicated, and reaches well into the subtle things in life like mood and everyday stress. Yet, this is the same infrastructure that can lead to pelvic and lower back pain when dysregulated.

3. Causes of Pelvic and Lower Back Pain

In addition to the conditions above, pelvic and lower back pain can be attributed to inflammation of the intra-abdomen and/or inflow (appendix and/or intestinal). All of these factors can be contributory when traumatologists treat people who walk through their door and say "when you do this" and "hurt here." Given the many contributors to the painful presentation of the pelvic area, the specific examination and diagnosis for each patient is undertaken only after a detailed interview of patient history.

- Bone and Soft Tissue refers to fractures, contusions, ligament sprains, and muscular strains. - Movement relates to both instantaneous strain (that particular last move you made) as well as repetitive strain. - Patho-anatomy is the result of a muscle, nerve, joint, or connective structure that was injured on a traumatic or macro-tiny level.

One of the biggest difficulties in treating pelvic and lower back pain is understanding where the pain is coming from and why the pain may occur today instead of yesterday. Overall, lower back and pelvic pain can come from three issues:

3.1. Musculoskeletal Causes

Muscles, bones, and connective tissues can contribute to pelvic or lower back pain. There are specific muscles and muscular areas that could be involved. Following is a list of the anatomical types of mechanisms that can cause symptoms: (A) Anatomical areas: (a) pelvis - innominate bone and pubic symphysis, (b) hip - acetabulum and other joint structures, and (c) lower back - structures that constitute the lumbar spine. (B) Muscles that can contribute: (a) deep low back and pelvic rotators, (b) abductor muscles, and (c) the iliotibial band and chronic minimus syndrome. The body's normal reaction to skeletal instability or abnormal loading patterns is to provide nervous system inhibitory signals to muscles in the same general area. Sometimes, as a result of this inhibitory process, different types of muscle imbalance can be created and may contribute to ongoing symptoms.

There are many areas in the human body that can contribute to or cause pelvic or lower back pain. Normally, the tendency is to think of organ malfunction or systemic disease processes as the originating cause, but other musculoskeletal and structural factors are commonly involved. These can be linked with either the anatomy of the bone framework where the pelvis and/or lower back form a part of, or could involve joint construction affecting the hips and/or the spine. Additionally, muscles and connective tissues (fascia, ligaments) are linked within the bony framework, and due to the expanse in surface area, these pain generators can influence others of the same nerve root levels and/or within the same neurological pathways.

3.2. Reproductive System Causes

The position of the uterus affecting back pain has also been researched in pregnancy, but there is currently no clear indication of any association. Lower back pain can be caused during or after pregnancy by ligaments being changed and the curving of the pelvis. A few women with mesh prolapses have reported lower back pain, which was resolved after surgery, implying that the prolapse can cause or worsen back pain. Pelvic pain in women is frequently the result of a problem with the female reproductive system, such as the fallopian tubes, ovaries, or lymph nodes, but not necessarily so. Swift et al. found that back pain was significantly more common in female patients with chronic pelvic pain than in controls and found that the greater the chronic pelvic pain, the more severe the back pain.

The uterus, ovaries, fallopian tubes, and vagina are contained in the pelvis and are referred to as below the pelvic diaphragm. The four positions of the uterus hold the uterus in place and are in the pelvis. The four positions are anteflexed, anteverted, retroflexed, and retroverted. While malpositioning of the uterus is widely thought to cause pelvic pain, there is little scientific evidence to support this theory. With endometriosis, uterine fibroids, or ovarian cysts, it is possible to feel a fullness in the pelvis. When inserting fingers in the vagina, painful nodules may commonly be felt in a patient with endometriosis. But one limitation to the node test is that it can increase the tone surrounding the muscle and cause fibroses. There are ultrasounds that can measure the size of the uterus, the size of the fibroids, and look for ovarian cysts. MRI scans are more precise than ultrasounds when looking into soft-tissue disease before surgery.

3.3. Gastrointestinal Causes

Relations between the digestive system and lower back pain provide healthcare professionals with valuable information about diagnosis and patient management. More research with larger sample sizes is necessary to explore these relationships further. Patients with symptoms of lower back pain commonly report abdominal and gastrointestinal symptoms, for example, constipation and diarrhea. Studies have shown that irritable bowel syndrome (IBS) is present in 28% of individuals with lower back pain. When individuals with back pain themselves were questioned in a recent study, 34% identified having digestive disorders, compared to 16% in the control group. Bowel diseases cause lower back pain and there is a relationship between spinal movement and gait disturbance as well as irritable bowel syndrome. When the compensation mechanism is impaired, there are feedback responses and, as a consequence, diseases of the lower back also cause dysfunction or disease in several organs including the digestive system. The causes of lower back pain can be divided into gastrointestinal and nutritional, urinary, tumors, endometriosis, gynecological, nerves, and infectious diseases.

Many anatomical features may explain the connection between the digestive tract and lower back pain, and these include blood supply, drug metabolism, digestion, immunity, signaling, and the nervous system. Movements of the lower spine may affect the digestive system and its processes or cause dysfunction because of the proximity of anatomical structures like nerves and blood vessels. Bowel diseases cause lower back pain in many individuals and result in dysfunction or disease in several organs including the nerves, causing referred pain. Prostaglandins, leukotrienes, interleukins, endorphins, and tumors in the digestive system additionally cause referred pain. There may be feedback between the digestive system and the lower back.

4. Diagnostic Approaches

Electrical tests measure speed down the nerve root, myelogram with and without CT examine the effect of pressure gradients on the nerve root, discography stretches the disc wall evaluating the progress of disc degeneration, and the electromyogram studies the electrical integrity of the muscles and the nerve root. Some of the tests used for visualizing pelvic pain include a systemic and somatic nerve conduction velocity test, partial motor speed test, pudendal terminal latency reflex test, measurement of the root evoked response during myelography, pelvic floor needle electromyography, high-resolution anal manometry, anal electromyography, proctography, and MRI. A selective nerve root block may also help a physician establish a diagnosis.

There are a variety of different approaches used to diagnose pelvic and lower back pain. These can include diagnostic blockade, x-ray, or fluoroscopy with discography, among many other methods. A physical therapy measurement of lumbar lordosis is often used by physicians as an in-office diagnostic test, while a posterior-anterior x-ray while lying down is especially useful as a diagnostic approach in the case of scoliosis. For adults, excessive flexion or extension of the lumbosacral spine can also be evaluated with hyperextension and hyperflexion x-rays, and custom sitting x-rays can show the effect of sitting on the load division between the lumbar discs. A direct x-ray of the thoracolumbar spine may show the extent of adult scoliosis. Some of the most useful tests for visualizing some cases of back pain are myelograms, CT scans, ultrasound of the nerve roots, high magnetic resonance imaging, bone scan, and radionuclide liquid scintigraphy.

4.1. Physical Examination

Changes in posture, vertical transfer mechanisms, and pain pattern may be elucidative for the clinician to determine the lumbopelvic origin of the symptoms. Insight into selecting posture, muscle activity, and vertical loading in relation to a lumbopelvic pain disorder can guide the clinician to accurately influence these factors in the treatment. Additionally, a rotational instability seems to play a role in chronic lumbopelvic pain. Core stability for lumbopelvic pain patients is necessary in performance tasks, such as going from a one leg stand to a two leg stand. For lumbopelvic pain patients in the rehabilitation phase, it can be recommended to begin with simple tasks and gradually increase the difficulty in combination with increasing the volume. This means that several times have to be trained successively before proceeding to, for instance, performing an One Leg Stand test on an Instable Power Plate.

Examinations, such as orthopedic and musculoskeletal tests, play a large role in diagnosing both pelvic and lumbosacral pain. Despite the increase in the use of imaging options, a working diagnosis is often created from the results of a physical assessment. The characteristics, including location and duration, of pelvic pain and low back pain overlap and share common sources. It was once believed that pelvic pain was a symptom of another disorder, such as lumbar spine disease; however, it is now thought to be a disorder in and of itself. In order to recognize and treat the symptoms of pelvic pain effectively,

the possibility for a confounding pain source must be
addressed.

4.2. Imaging Studies

Magnetic resonance imaging (MRI) is a preferred initial test to identify the source of pain as it can help detect pathology in the cortical bone, medulla and bone marrow, neural elements, and paraspinous muscle that IBD may influence. Bone scans are done to exclude spinal metastases, pseudoarthroses, and spondylitis from the decreased bone density linked to IBD or osteoporosis. Gallium scans are sensitive in identifying a number of bacterial, fungal, and parasitic infections. Determining the nature of the infection is possible with good interreader accuracies among experienced readers, but the utility and possibility of interreader agreement in spondylodiscitis are unknown. Finally, differentiation of a degenerative anterior spondylolisthesis from an isthmic spondylolisthesis on MRI and CT is unnecessary, as it has no impact on vertebral augmentation.

There are a wide variety of imaging studies that can be used to evaluate the causes of pelvic and lower back pain. X-rays allow visualization of the anatomic structures of the lumbar spine, including assessment of disc space height, osteophytes, facet joint space, and gross assessment of the vertebrae and possible fractures. Annotated X-rays can demonstrate evidence of previous lumbar cage surgery, with the appearance of laminectomies and fusion. Myelography is performed by injecting a small amount of contrast material into the cerebrospinal fluid (the fluid that surrounds the spinal cord and nerves) to detect abnormal development, tumors, and other problems linked to increased pressure in the brain. A computed tomography (CT) scan allows for the visualization of the lumbar spine in a cross-section to detect bone injury or narrowing of the spinal canal associated with tumors or herniated intervertebral discs, among other problems.

Imaging Studies: No Level (e.g. CADRE)

4.3. Laboratory Tests

Some authors have suggested that laboratory tests can give important information, i.e. possible structural abnormality of a disc or possible involvement of nerve root in the compression, but these conclusions based on logical deduction. X-ray provides actual anatomical structures of the vertebras, and CT (Computer tomography) is more appropriate in diagnosis of the source of pain, i.e. discopathy or stenosis of the canalis vertebralis. If these results are found, LBP itself cannot be invalidated. Such a process also goes for MRI with the advantage of no irradiation. Sciatica is differentiated from simple LBP based on clinical symptoms. Each of them, X-ray, CT, and MRI, is not sufficient to diagnose LBP accurately. On the other hand, laboratory tests sometimes give misleading information. Blood biochemical tests will guide meaningful remedies and some are used for the follow-up. If a doctor gains meaningful results of high blood pressure from taking blood pressure, he or she will prescribe a drug to decrease the blood pressure. He or she can check its effectiveness through taking blood pressure again, not through examining the structures of blood vessels. Even if positive results of X-ray and/or CT and MRI are revealed for LBP, (obviously it does not always occur) the importance of structures belong into attention is controversial. There are subjective symptoms and subjective complaints also. If an obtained pain-controlled period through appropriate measures is long regardless findings on X-ray, for example, a poor association between the structure of lumbar vertebra and LBP is suggested from these findings.

It is sensible to use tests if we have acknowledged some continuous relations. If these tests could demonstrate a low relationship with the condition of subjects, they will be considered as insensible tests. But if they are sensitive, a strong association may exist between variations of the laboratory tests and the level of pain. Nowadays, laboratory tests are widely used in the research of the LBP. They are used to detect the source of complaints and sometimes used for planning and follow-up the progress. Blood biochemical are valid in the diagnoses of some syndromes, i.e. infectious diseases, malignancy, hormonal and metabolic disorders. Since the nature of LBP does not belong to these diseases, the role of the laboratory tests still need to be identified.

5. Treatment Options

There are three types of treatments currently available for chronic lower back pain: medication, interventional procedures, and physical interventions. Both types of medication are aimed at reducing pain perception and are supported by some evidence demonstrating their effectiveness. Spinal, sacroiliac joint, and major nerve blocks directly focus on the secondary causes of pain. Lastly, invasive treatments such as surgery and neurostimulation directly target the primary causes of lower back pain. All of these treatment methods are viable options for some patients, whereas for others, their ability to be treated may be reduced. While many aspects of the mechanisms behind physical interventions remain controversial, they are among the most commonly recommended treatments. These treatments help to make individuals who have lower back pain less likely to experience disability, and the majority of those living with chronic pain due to lower back problems get better.

The treatment options available for chronic pain in the lower back and pelvic region are numerous, offering multiple opportunities to treat these conditions in a variety of settings. Many of these options are directly targeted at one of the secondary causes of pain previously described. Before discussing the evidence behind these treatment options, we present a list of available treatments and their mechanisms.

5.1. Conservative Therapies

In conclusion, pain is not easily compartmentalized, and the brain's perception of a painful stimulus can be influenced by the interpretation of that stimulus within the spinal cord and within the higher brain regions. Muscle, which is richly innervated in the lower back and pelvic region, can not only produce pain because of the activity of the nociceptive (pain) nerve endings, but the muscle receptors can change in behavior and influence the sensory receptors in the back and pelvis and the association centers of the brain to initiate a pain signal. The combination of all these receptors and feelings can produce LBP, LPP, and BNLP. Even though muscle pain can be created by nociceptive input, once the nociceptive input is gone, the perception of pain can be long-lasting. This explains why there may be a relationship between a silent spine, without nociceptor activity post-surgically, and no relief from LBP.

Given the patient populations discussed in the previous sections, it is clear that the first phases of care for a patient with symptoms of the PGP, the PN, the LBP, the LPP, and the LBNP should be focused on conservative treatments. There are a number of non-invasive, non-surgical treatments that are undertaken in an effort to improve these LPP/LBP symptoms before medications and surgery are considered. Bodywork or body-mechanics approaches carried out by a physical or manual therapist can help address movement impairments and muscle flexibility and strength limitations that can be related to PGP and PN symptoms.

5.2. Medications

There is no study that promotes the "ideal" medication management protocol for pelvic pain. Pelvic pain has been usually studied as primary dysmenorrhea, secondary dysmenorrhea, or adjuvant painful conditions, with very few studies performed on CPP. In patients with low back pain associated with reproductive issues, Painful Bladder Syndrome/Interstitial Cystitis (PBS/IC) showed pain relief by using amitriptyline, which is used as an antidepressant with analgesic effects. However, this study did not directly evaluate amitriptyline as isolated primary medication for low back pain associated with pelvic condition.

In clinical practice, various studies recommend different medications. In a systematic review, Keller et al. recommended different medications based on the causes of pelvic pain. Gonzalez Casas et al. suggest that in cancer patients with low back pain, a combination of acetaminophen and opioids is better than ibuprofen in terms of pain control reduction when first-line treatment with paracetamol or ibuprofen does not work, replacing them with opioids. Petra et al. argue that when primary dysmenorrhea is very severe, patients can use a combination of paracetamol and non-steroidal anti-inflammatory drugs (NSAIDs) for pain relief. Since low back pain is usually a combination of nociceptive and neuropathic mechanisms, medications target both types of pain. NSAIDs work as a primary option for inflammation (pure nociceptive pain) and pain control. In contrast to low back pain, pelvic pain, especially chronic pain, presents prominent neuropathic pain in the background. Therefore, reproductive pelvic pain may show a good response to pregabalin, a neuropathic pain targeted oral agent. While acetaminophen is usually recommended as a combined analgesic with opioids, some guidelines suggest adding it from the beginning as paracetamol has a weak central effect and it is believed it can reduce the amount of opioid required. Patients should use NSAIDs for only short periods due to a higher risk of ulcer and risks to the cardiovascular system and kidneys.

Pharmacological Management

5.3. Surgical Interventions

1. Microdiscectomy—within the past three years, researchers have indicated that oral steroids and epidural steroids have limited to no consistent results on the relief of lower back pain. A microdiscectomy could be called for if the pain has lasted over a year, but it is imperative to ensure patients are not prematurely foisted into surgery. Many patients endure the pain of their herniation and enjoy a moderate increase in their ability to walk within just six weeks' time. A significant improvement in overall back pain could also occur. The electrical signals moving from the stressful lower spine to the muscles generally reach near-normal levels after three months. This is considered a significant period for the patient in terms of their healing.

More invasive methods for dealing with lower back pain are in the realm of neurosurgery. The primary aim of these surgeries is to reduce the amount of pain an individual feels by separating problematic areas. Unlike the treatments earlier in the paper, surgical interventions do not necessarily and directly treat pelvic pain, but they are performed when individuals have such severe or refractory pain originating in the lower back that less invasive treatments are ineffective. Some of these methods are warranted only in cases where individuals have lost control of some aspect of their lower bowel or bladder, due to redundancies in the nervous system. Other surgeries are more typically indicated to address severe lower back pain that is the result when people have physical redundancy that increases the amount of pressure on certain parts of the spinal region.

6. Preventive Strategies

A Chinese study showed that overweight adult patients benefited from a reduction in body weight. Findings in the literature for overweight or obese children's relationship with back pain have been inconsistent. Prevention is important to prevent recurrence and chronic pain. For prevention, all conservative, non-drug treatments and lifestyle recommendations are important, alleviate acute or persistent pain subacute, and improve quality of life. Protect yourself against pelvic and lower back pain with these preventive strategies: 1) Avoid overuse; 2) Use ergonomics; 3) Use proper body mechanics; 4) Bend without pain; 5) Lift properly; 6) Keep a strong core; 7) Exercise to maintain good bone health.

Pelvic and lower back pain may be a result of harmful factors. Several strategies may be viewed not only as a way to manage pain but also as a strategy to prevent it. Those strategies are: avoidance of muscle overuse related to static positions, appropriate body mechanics during activities involving lifting heavy items, proper bending techniques, appropriate lifting techniques, weight management/reduction, core muscle strength, and aerobic exercise. It can be concluded that there is enough evidence to support most preventive strategies. People carrying excess weight have a higher risk of developing chronic low back pain, but there is not a convincing link between body mass index and acute low back pain. Core muscle exercises

with aerobic and flexibility exercises can reduce low back
pain.

6.1. Exercise and Physical Activity

Other physical experiences, such as occupational activities, are also linked with pelvic floor dysfunctions and low back pain. However, little evidence links activity level with musculoskeletal low back pain in non-pregnant young and middle-aged women. It appears that physical activities in general are beneficial in preventing pelvic pain. More studies should be conducted to examine the relationship between regular physical activities and the development of these pains. Low back pain is a major cause of disability. Patients are frequently advised to cease sports and physical activities that provoke pain because it has long been assumed that exercise increases the risk of future low back pain. However, more recent findings suggest that regular physical activity has protective effects, including a decreased risk at the level of the lower back during daily life activities and leisure time sports. Therefore, lack of exercise may lead to a decrease in lumbar musculature and control, thereby increasing the risk. To examine the relationship between physical activity and low back pain, four cohort studies were conducted. The results showed that low physical activity levels increased the risk of low back pain, while moderate to high physical activity levels reduce the risk.

Having a physically active life is beneficial, as exercising has been proved to prevent the prevalence of pelvic and lower back pain. Pelvic pain is significantly associated with a lower frequency of regular exercise among pregnant women, but it is not clear whether increased physical activity would decrease lower back pain during pregnancy or not. A meta-analysis suggests a potential effect of tai chi in the improvement of pelvic pain during pregnancy, but more experiments are needed to examine the relationship between regular exercise and the occurrence of pelvic pain.

6.2. Ergonomics and Posture

Good posture alone does not have a great effect on increasing work productivity and decreasing musculoskeletal discomfort when sitting. The work area and its physical design can greatly affect how the body can be positioned. For effective pain control, people also need to modify their environment so that they can assume beneficial postures. Increasing the amount of contact between a work area's design and an individual's body makes for distributed loading of weight with decreased contact stress, resulting in decreased muscle action. Managing posture also requires an individual to work with his or her workplace to minimize awkward postures through changes in position and movement.

Ergonomics involves the design of the environment according to the posture and proportions of the body. It helps people to work efficiently without harming themselves. For those sitting for prolonged periods, the chair is the most important. Posture is equally important for reducing or eliminating pelvic and lower back pain. It is the way in which a body is held or carried while sitting or standing. When the chair and a person's posture are correct, the body is positioned to work more effectively and comfortably. Additionally, there is often an enhanced chance that the person will not have pain that starts in the pelvis or lower back. In this article, ergonomics and posture management are described and explored further.

7. Psychosocial Factors in Pelvic and Lower Back Pain

To understand the relationship between psychosocial factors and complaints of pain in the pelvic area and/or lower back, it is first of all necessary to understand what the pelvis is and how it works (the anatomy and physiology of the pelvic region). Even more important is the fact that the pelvis is part of the body of a human and not only a mass of bones, joints, and muscles. (This means that psychological and social factors that are related to both the pelvis and the rest of the body are explored in parallel in the following subsections.) If the pelvis is seen to be a part of the body, then it is necessary to take other parts of the body into account as well. If someone goes to see a doctor with complaints about pain in the pelvis, the social relations with or the psychological functioning of the rest of the body are not necessarily considered. Therefore, the other parts of the body are not represented in this state-of-the-art article.

Quite a few studies have explored how psychosocial and social factors are related to pain in the pelvic area or the lower back, or both. Two systematic reviews concluded that there was moderate evidence for a relationship with emotional abuse and a belief in a genetic predisposition to disease. A protective factor may be knowing about anatomical structures. Quality of life and work dissatisfaction were also related to a diagnosis of chronic pelvic pain. Additional literature shows that there are many other psychological or social factors related to chronic pelvic or back pain. Some of the problems are even more strongly related to chronic pain in the pelvic area than they are to chronic pain in the lower back. These additional factors are explored in the subsections below.

7.1. Stress and Pain Perception

Repeated stress is a common factor contributing to the development of several pelvic pains but differs with the emotion and intensity of stress-induced pelvic pain. In addition, stress targets the same pelvic region and blood vessels to contribute to psychological burden and pelvic pain, which may form the stress-pain relationships. The pelvis serves many important functions, including housing and protecting reproductive organs and the excretory and reproductive tracts. It also provides essential body support as well as having sexual and communicative functions. However, few theories exist to assess the pain and biomechanics of both the pelvic organs and lumbar spine.

Stress and pain perception: The relationship between psychological stress and pelvic and lower back pain perception is clearer. While psychological stress preferentially contributes to the experience of lower back pain, it also contributes to pelvic pain. The relationship between psychological stress increases and causes an increase in reported pelvic and lower back pain. While reports of pelvic pain decreased after a period of time, the pelvic pain symptom severity remained directly associated with perceived stress. This is in contrast with reported decreases in low back pain intensity after the period of stress. To conclude, recent scientific evidence suggests complex interactions between stress and the brain mechanisms modulating the perception of pelvic versus low back pain. The results suggest a bidirectional interaction between structural brain changes and the severity of self-reported pelvic pain during psychological stress. A ministroke in our brain, which may be too small to notice clinically, can activate higher processing centers in our brain to change their resting patterns of activity, which in turn leads to altered responses to stressful stimuli. Only the resting changes in brain activity in response to stress can either increase or decrease the severity of our pelvic pain, but not both.

7.2. Psychological Interventions

The flow model of pain suggests that pain perception is influenced by sensory, cognitive, and emotional inputs. This allows us to modulate pain through psychological interventions such as cognitive-behavioral therapy (CBT), acceptance and commitment therapy (ACT), mindfulness, education, and qi gong with the aim of reducing pain and improving psychological well-being. Long-term follow-ups are needed to determine the exact lasting effects of pain management on not just a rehabilitation outcome such as pain, but pain and the biopsychosocial areas. Given the best available evidence, collaborative psychological and medical management is advised to treat symptoms of serial abuse that continue despite resolution of physical symptoms. There needs to be alternative engagement strategies to best improve psychiatric symptoms and reduce disability in individuals who either categorically refuse, are unable to, or cannot, for patient safety considerations, entertain pharmacologic options. The best management strategy is dependent on the individual patient, their family, their healthcare providers, and the investigative, regulatory, and patient management policies of the local community.

Psychological approaches have the potential to reduce perceptions of pain and improve psychological well-being. Acceptance and Commitment Therapy (ACT) is a form of CBT that focuses on reducing the impact of the thoughts and feelings associated with pain. Research investigating ACT to reduce pain and improve function in people with pelvic girdle pain has shown promising signs. Depression is a term often used to broadly describe a worsening in mental well-being and mental health. An estimated 60-90% of people with chronic lower back pain report clinically significant depression. Cognitive Behavioural Therapy (CBT) is designed to treat behavioral and thought patterns; current research about CBT shows that it is a good tool to help people improve depression and anxiety. Mindfulness moves away from challenging the negative thought as it does with CBT and instead involves accepting your thoughts and feelings. Two studies have shown that pain intensity didn't change, however, people reported less disability. This implies that mindfulness-based therapies do not change the pain per se, but it does allow people to live their lives and complete activities that are important to them. QiGong is another form of pain coping strategy, focusing on deep breathing and light exercises; it warrants further research to determine its effects on pain and function.

8. Special Considerations for Women

Two studies from Brazil suggest that proximal vagal (splenic) function is depressed in sufferers of chronic pelvic pain, while two studies on irritable bowel syndrome (IBS) suggest there is no difference in depressed cardiopulmonary vagal tone relative to healthy controls. All studies of chronic pelvic pain or IBS relative to asymptomatic controls suggest that self-reported heart rate variability (HRV) is more depressed in chronic pelvic pain and/or IBS sufferers, and this may be related to the severity of their symptoms. A more global index of the balance between the autonomic nervous system's splanchnic (gut) versus cardiac (heart) branches could be derived via a basic test of heart rate - the response to an exhale-inhale ratio change. This ratio may be a valuable comparison measure as chronic pelvic pain perturbation may not be segregated to basic regulation differences in only the gut (as tested in heart rate-to-breathing studies), but may be more global to all vagal-cardiac regulation.

In a 2015 research review, it was suggested that female pelvic pain may manifest differently from that in men. Meanwhile, chronic pelvic pain may also be more common among women than men, especially involving pelvic organs. Given the higher lifetime prevalence of low-back pain, chronic pelvic pain, and the fact that many of the same organs involved in chronic pelvic pain (e.g., bladder, vagina, uterus) sit near low-back pain-generating structures, special consideration of these issues in women is necessary.

8.1. Pregnancy-Related Pain

Thus, this study aimed to evaluate the prevalence of lumbar pain and radiculopathy or sciatica concomitantly with hip complaints in the immediate postpartum period, as well as to determine the primary affected radicular distribution related to hip pain more frequently associated with a lower back condition.

Although classified as two different complaints, hip or pelvic girdle pain is frequently associated with mechanical dysfunctions of the lumbosacral spine. When they occur together, they compromise the overall function and quality of life of the suffering subjects. The prevalence of the complaints varies depending on the criteria used for diagnosis and ranges in the literature between 5 and 9% of the cases when considering just pelvic or hip pain, with the majority of studies finding that the pain is more prevalent during the second trimester of pregnancy. When considering radicular complaints originating from the lower back, the prevalence varies between 1 and 1.71% on the same side opposite to the hip complaints. The literature on the subject is nil when considering the symptoms during the immediate postpartum period.

In April 1980, the term "PGP" (pelvic girdle pain) replaced the council Parietal to be able to identify the pelvic region from the reference to uterine pain causes in patients with endometriosis that until that time were the main reason women sought health services. This same classification was ratified in 1984 and also used in the proponents' daily clinical practice.

Pregnancy-related pelvic girdle pain (PGP) and lower back pain (LBP) are common issues experienced by many pregnant individuals. Regarding the pelvic or musculoskeletal pain, it is important to clarify that it generally appears as the pregnancy progresses, causing physical discomfort, limitations in physical activity, loss of muscle tone in those who've been pregnant, mood changes, and/or sleep disorders.

8.2. Menstrual Cycle and Pain

Hormonal influence, particularly the experience of and changes during menses and menstruation, could be associated with the development of pain in living with PPC. However, there is a dearth of information available. Nevertheless, hormonal fluctuations during the menstrual cycle have been shown to be associated with alterations in the stress and pain experience in non-pain groups. Pain experience is also influenced by the phase of the menstrual cycle, with testosterone reaching a nadir paralleling menstrual estrogen and progesterone levels during the onset of menses, when levels of cortisol increase in response to the local inflammatory markers present. Despite a lack of information specifically in PPP or CPP patients, the data indicate the influence of the menstrual cycle phase on stress pathways and the pain experience in non-pain groups. Interestingly, anterior cruciate ligament injuries have been found to occur most frequently in the follicular phase, implying that stabilizers of the lumbopelvic musculature may also be under increased tension. Phase-related hormonal influence on premenstrual pelvic floor muscle tension or cramping (primary dysmenorrhea) in women could potentially lead to hypothalamic-pituitary-adrenal axis activation, and tension changing nociceptor thresholds and, in some cases, contribute to increased pain in PPC or CPP.

There is little direct research on the relationship between the menstrual cycle and possible changes in the associations or influence on comorbid back pain with pelvic pain conditions. While women have been found to have a 1% greater lifetime risk of developing chronic pelvic pain than men, the presentation of low back pain is otherwise similar between the sexes. The majority of studies that have examined the relationship between pelvic pain (musculoskeletal or visceral) and comorbid low back pain report adjustments for sex, but these data are not presented or denoted in published manuscripts. However, in one prospective cohort of spinal pain patients (PronteSPIN), women with a 'lumbopelvic' pain distribution presented with the same number of manual musculoskeletal pain areas as men and were found to be at no greater risk of psychological distress. Of these studies, the majority report illness or disease whereas only seven noted pain, and of these, only two reported menstrual data, finding that twinges, knots, and pain were worst the day before and the first day of menstruation post-hysterectomy, or in the second week of the menstrual cycle.

9. Impact of Age and Lifestyle

A patient's lifestyle and occupation must also be considered, as prolonged or unaccustomed loads on the lower back and pelvis can induce pain and overload in the surrounding myotenofascial tissue. Prolonged sitting and sedentary lifestyles can change posture, promote muscle inhibition or atrophy and lead to decreased physical capacity. Decreased physical capacity can in turn lead to changes in lower limb mechanics and increased pelvis, sacrum or lumbar spine movement, which can subsequently lead to pain and injury. Endpoints such as one-sided pain, concomitant pain, single registration of infection and data linked to the classification of pain on a VAS score.

Pelvic and lower back pain has increasingly been targeted by researchers and healthcare professionals in recent years. Based on the authors' own clinical expertise, it is often unclear what is the primary driver of symptoms, the lower back or the pelvic region. More often than not, both the lower back and the pelvis are sources of a patient's pain and require management. Pathoanatomical relationships between the pelvis and lower back have also been found, which could explain the higher incidence of concomitant pain between the pelvis and lumbar spine region. This section aims to understand how age and lifestyle impact the pelvis and lower back region, as these factors may lead to both local and regional pain syndromes. Patients in the older age groups often present with concomitant lower back and pelvic pain, as degenerative and traumatic changes can affect more than one region of the body.

9.1. Pediatric Population

In line with a previous study on an adult population, summarizing the most frequently experienced pain in populations similar to those of our young patients, then 39% of the subjects reported injury to the lumbar segments with symptoms located strictly in the pelvis, and 12.3% with the presence of bilaterally combined lumbar and inguinal symptoms. These findings suggest that even if inguinal injuries associated with lumbosacral injuries are present in the pediatric population, the underlying neurological causes are looked at in a different way. Pediatric consultation studies of sports and early-liver disease provide further support for the above findings on the appropriate interpretation of inguinal injuries in children. Our findings regarding pelvic injuries in children are consistent with Waldron's reports of the features of degenerative diseases at different ages between the cartilage and the talus.

First and foremost, as children grow and develop, their turning, which has already been mentioned in the previous sections related to the adult population, is also more unevenly distributed. Since the average adult's TI position is around 2, the painful sensations experienced by the children occurring in the location of the first lumbar segment suggest further research of the relationship between these locations in children. Exactly 50% of our study population reported painful sensations suddenly radiating from the lower back to the pelvis, in the form of acute lumbosacral pain both in the left and right inguinal areas. This could be interpreted as an injury to the distal termination of the spinal process, present in the first lumbar, and in exactly the middle, even before it enters the pelvis. In fact, this segment processes these sensitive qualities, and such a pathological condition, which directly and suddenly activates the sinking of nociceptive impulses to this level, has no place in congestive fibrosis lesions. Such information can be useful in verifying which way to turn when planning to further develop neuropathic pain in children.

9.2. Geriatric Population

There are numerous lifestyle changes that must be accounted for, including whether an individual can drive or needs assistance in transportation, as well as economic difficulties and inadequate medical insurance. Elders also tend to have mental and emotional concerns, such as a low quality of life, stress, alcohol abuse, and poor nutrition, which can influence the individual's mind, emotional stress, social help support, and the backing of family and friends. There are particular women-specific musculoskeletal risk factors, including lower bone density, contraceptive utilization, and aging-related hormonal changes. Different from youngsters, intra-abdominal strength is an important factor regarding the aging of the pelvic floor. To sum up, the pelvic and low back area are not isolated, but a functioning musculoskeletal system that might be influenced by influences other than those of the skeletal muscles and tissues. The low back and the pelvis are foundations, a region of mechanical stability that is a necessity for the pelvis. They are affected by both the bodily and functional effects of the aging process.

9.2. Geriatric population: Aging is defined by progressive changes in body physiology and body morphology, which also extend to pelvic and lower back pain. As a result, both pelvic and lower back pain are major health-related complaints in the elderly. The worldwide estimate is approximately 30%, with reports drawn from higher proportions and greater amounts of pelvic floor and generalized pain. According to the clinical guidelines set by the American College of Physicians and the American Pain Society for lower back pain, it is estimated that the symptoms of low back pain persist or recur in the elderly. Moreover, older adults have diminished homeostasis and lower sensory and motor performance, which can have a direct negative effect on treatment efficacy. They also tend to have multiple long-term comorbidities, a higher number of medications, decreased responses to interventions, and an augmented degree of caution, all of which can impact the relationship with healthcare providers and therapists.

10. Emerging Research and Therapies

One entity that is now benefiting from emerging research and therapies is women with post-partum sacral pain. Sacral pain levels and patient function have received considerably less scientific scrutiny when compared to other low back structures, but one new study has determined that four out of five women undergoing epidural or ethylcellulose injections for persistent PGP rated their symptoms as "significantly improved" and those rated improvements were maintained at 3 months. As practitioners in most areas, surgical and manual therapies may not be our first-line defense for a musculoskeletal complaint. The natural and high-level mechanisms in place to protect the left knee or lumbosacral spine are invaluable. Protective mechanisms can run awry and cause symptoms, though - especially in an injured runner who continues to run. And the intent in surgery or manual care is not to take the pain away "just because it's there," but to more safely utilize those protective mechanisms as the person returns to sport/activity.

In the realm of pelvic, lumbar, and sacral pain and rehabilitation, many are excited about emerging, long-awaited research that has occurred and, moreover, the anatomic relationships that are beginning to be elucidated between pelvic floor dysfunction and lumbar and sacral elements. While surgeons and manual therapists have seen longstanding anecdotes confirming that rehabilitating one region can help improve pain and function in the other, researchers are just now beginning to concretely demonstrate the structural relationships between the pelvic floor and the lower back.

10.1. Biomechanical Innovations

Given the amount of research focusing on the lumbo-pelvic-hip complex, highlighted are the articles focusing on pelvic dysfunction that contribute to or result from pain in the pelvic and/or low back region. The articles are intended to be directly relevant to the treatment of these patients and will review the effectiveness of novel and time-tested medicines and interventions, and give insight into the future directions that will benefit personal and physical therapy. The emerging healthcare market related to such pelvic and/or lower back pain includes "wearables" designed to monitor alignment and other forces or aspects of human movement in an effort to prevent injuries or promote well-being. Given the importance of the relationship between the pelvis and lower limb movement, its importance in rehabilitating patients with musculoskeletal disorders, and the emergence of commercial technologies to stimulate the pelvis and muscles attached to it, the potential future treatment in orthopedics has broad importance.

The underlying goal of this research topic is to display some of the newest innovations in the biomechanical realm. The interactions between the pelvic and lower back regions are critical to our understanding of many different forms of musculoskeletal pain. The four articles contained in this section begin with an examination of the relationship between pelvic and low back pain in two studies assessing lateral lumbo-pelvic muscle activity during slow and fast-paced walking. We then delve into a targeted overview of the back pain and potential future treatments in a focus article discussing randomized controlled trials on intervertebral discs and the lumbar multifidus in patients with low back pain.

10.2. Mind-Body Approaches

Biologically, the systems that activate the stress response (the HPA axis and the autonomic nervous system's sympathetic branch) also play a critical role in modulating many systems involved in pain signaling (for example, the signals from A-delta and C fibers in the peripheral nervous system, the processing of ascending pain signals in the spinal cord, and descending modulation of pain perception in the brain). If pain and these stress systems continue to be activated over an extended period of time, pain processing can change in ways that make pain persist even in the absence of the initial injury. Current research is seeking to determine the optimal parameters for mind-body interventions for pelvic and LS pain presentations, how to best integrate them with other more mechanically-based treatments, and how to identify which patients are most likely to benefit from their use. There is also emerging interest in the potential of more socially-based therapeutic modalities that recognize the psychosocial interconnectedness of patients with inter-related pelvic and lower back pain conditions.

In general, mind-body therapies aim to engage brain pathways that contribute to relaxation and stress relief. These techniques are often referred to as "holistic therapies" and may include taking a mind-body approach trip to sessions. Psychotherapeutic approaches that have been studied for people with chronic pelvic or lower back pain include biofeedback, relaxation training, hypnosis, and psychoeducation based on biopsychosocial and/or fear-avoidance models of pain presentation. A detailed description of each of these interventions is beyond the scope of this publication, though readers can find details about them within the original article by Fritz et al.

11. Conclusion and Future Directions

When isolated, subjects with pelvic dysfunction showed an observable change in coordination, despite previously being asymptomatic. However, in this young, healthy population, area showed significant differences in pelvic tendon vibration in addition to six subjects, which indicated atypical lack of coordination between the upper and lower pelvic system. These levels of atypical pelvic control paradox, dominant, and non-dominant lower extremities for problems associated with gait and lumbopelvic movement, including the potential connections to SAM. The underlying spinal control and relationship with SAM remain to be explored. The findings of this study set the stage for investigating pelvic control in impaired populations who have dynamic lumbopelvic instability, or with an increased risk for low back pain, including but not relegated to females after childbirth (with diastasis rectus abdominus, lumbopelvic pain, etc.), postpartum, and athletes such as dancers and runners.

Synchronizing the spinal, pelvic, and lower limb joints is an essential feature of human walking. Pain or joint pathology in any of these joints may disrupt normal walking patterns and result in redistribution of movement or number of steps, causing a compensatory motion at other joints. Defining the primary cause of a patient's pain can be difficult since believed causes may be associated with pelvic or sacroiliac joint dysfunction or a referred pain master source by the ligament, muscles, or nerves innervating the lumbosacral spine. Current literature has shown that pelvic rotation could alter normal hamstring and gluteus muscle activity in cases of low back pain. Although our results did not show altered hamstring activity as measured by muscle length, subjects with pelvic dysfunction did have reduced gluteal muscle activity and peak torque of the knee extensors. It is not clear why the literature reported increased EMG responses in these muscles as the subject presented with low back pain while our study did not.

The Comprehensive Guide to Managing Pelvic and Lower Back Pain

1. Introduction to Pelvic and Lower Back Pain

The goal of this paper is to provide you with a comprehensive guide to managing pelvic and lower back pain. The goal of this essay is to give you a general overview of back pain and pelvic pain, as well as an overview of associated diseases. In this straightforward essay, treatments and considerations are also discussed. To keep this information as general as possible, we will not discuss the cause and effects of back pain and pelvic pain specifically caused by a comorbidity such as endometriosis or musculoskeletal disorders.

While almost everybody has an episode of lower back pain at some point, the exact cause is hard to discern given the number of structures and body systems in the lower back. The majority of the time, the diagnosis can be based on a careful patient history and physical examination. Therapy is directed at the suspected pathophysiology of the affected person. Drug therapy depends on whether the pain is chronic or acute. Furthermore, as appropriate, nonpharmacologic alternatives are frequently helpful. Efforts for self-care and long-term therapy are often useful. Pelvic pain can be caused by a variety of diseases or illnesses. Management of pelvic pain typically involves drug treatment, physical therapy, psycho-regulation, or other therapeutic methods.

Pelvic and lower back pain affects each person at some point for several reasons. It does not usually cause a great deal of injury. The causes of pelvic pain and lower back issues vary. Pain management needs to be comprehensive. It includes drug therapy, physical activity, and stress control.

2. Understanding the Anatomy and Causes of Pelvic and Lower Back Pain

The pelvic region is made up of the sacrum, hip bones or innominate (and inside them are the ischium, ilium, and pubis), and two more bones - the coccyx or tailbone, and the femurs. Stretching of the lower back for an extended period of time or lifting/pushing objects can cause pelvic instability with soft tissue injury. Four main causes of pelvic pain are pelvic girdle pain, nerve pain, sacroiliac joint pain, and piriformis syndrome. The back is made up of three sections: the cervical spine, thoracic spine, and lumbar spine. The former originates at the base of the skull and goes down to the top of the scapula. Thoracic vertebrae connect to the anterior clavicle. The lumbar spine or lower back occupies the central position of the 3. Rates of lower back pain begin to rise in the 2nd to 4th decades and are associated with posture and occupational biomechanical demands. It can be divided into both axial and radicular types and may arise from disc degeneration, muscle strain, or an assortment of other potential musculoskeletal injuries. Types of lower back pain and their prevalence may differ between laborers and surgical candidates. Without delving deeply into medical jargon surrounding biomechanics and pain, it is feasible to say lower back pain has multifactorial etiologies. Non-specific causes are thought to be primarily musculoskeletal, with disc and facet joint pathologies being the most common.

The pelvic and lower back regions are infamous for causing pain in a plethora of individuals. In fact, the prevalence of low back pain related to the pelvic region is thought to range between 14% and 59%. Such a large range is due to the fact that management and understanding the etiology of chronic pelvic pain and radicular pain that may have its origin involving pelvic structures is difficult. It's critical that an explanation of potential pain generators in these regions begins with an understanding of the structures that comprise the pelvic and lumbar spine areas.

3. Common Conditions Leading to Pelvic and Lower Back Pain

To simplify the discussion, causes of pelvic and lower back pain can be grouped into four categories: musculoskeletal causes, gynecological causes, urological causes, and digestive causes. Musculoskeletal causes of pelvic and lower back pain are often the most manageable among the four categories. Degenerative joint or disc disease may result in the narrowing of the neural foramina and lead to radicular pain in the L5-SI distribution or sacroiliac joint pain. Very rarely, nerve root pain in the distribution above L5 is experienced. Back pain with radicular pain extending below the knee is referred to as sciatica. Sacroiliac joint pain can be differentiated from a herniated intervertebral disc or nerve root impingement by moving the joint, which worsens pain in the case of the sacroiliac joint.

A myriad of conditions may lead to pelvic and lower back pain, which typically result from either a musculoskeletal or non-musculoskeletal etiology. Among the most common causes are osteoarthritis and other conditions leading to mechanical back pain, urinary tract infections, and menstrual pain. Differentiating among these conditions can be difficult for some clinicians and individuals, although with a detailed history and evaluation, not only can the source of pelvic pain be determined, but appropriate steps can be taken to prevent future occurrences. Additionally, lower back pain may result from neural compression, a condition that is rapidly becoming more common in an increasingly overweight and obese population that is engaged in little physical activity.

3.1. Musculoskeletal Causes

Pain in the musculoskeletal system may originate not only from bones, joints, ligaments, and tendons, but also from the muscles themselves. There is also another way in which non-nervous problems such as muscular, ligamentous, bony, joint, or mechanical pains in other parts of the body can result in referred pain in the lower back, pelvis, or genitalia, and might be mistaken for prostatitis or other pelvic diseases. Dysfunction in the musculoskeletal system not only causes pain but can also contribute to functional disorders such as walking and sexual dysfunction. From a clinical perspective, the functions and pains of muscles, fascia, bones, and joints are closely interconnected. Changes in one of these structures, such as growth, spasm, or disintegration, can lead to unfavorable patterns in the others, and persistent pain and/or inflammation in muscles can affect sensorimotor control and limit joint range of motion and functionality. Conversely, excessive workload and musculoskeletal pain can result in reduced functional capacity, leading to further pain. In some diseases, vulvar pain and muscle pain can not only coexist but also exacerbate each other. Fascia is another structure that has received more attention in pain literature in recent years. The role of fasciae in creating and transmitting pain occurs not only through nerves but also due to fascial-skeletal or myofascial structures. Muscles do not just attach to distinct locations on the bones; they also have an impact on functionality beyond what is expected. Overall, these systems are highly interconnected.

In the context of pelvic pain, it is suitable to give credit to the muscles, bones, and joints, which form the musculoskeletal system and are the most relevant to healthcare professionals in their daily practice. This chapter attempts to create an imaginary matrix of these accessory structures, in order to provide an understanding of the anatomical connections that facilitate healthcare practice. However, we can only hope for a skeleton of information rather than a complete structure. Conceptually focusing on musculoskeletal causes and related pains is extremely difficult due to the presence of multiple health conditions and the multidimensional nature of pelvic pain. Pelvic pain is often described as mechanical, musculoskeletal, somatic, somatic-tropic, and/or nociceptive in nature. We prefer to discuss these pains as an association. Additionally, categorizing pelvic and/or low back pain conditions strictly as musculoskeletal is controversial.

3.2. Gynecological Causes

The gynecological aspect should be taken into account in order to form a more comprehensive approach and differential diagnosis for pelvic and/or low back pain—in women only and among other possible causes (such as vascular and urologic). The differential diagnosis for various gynecological diseases presenting with low back pain can be quite difficult, therefore the gynecologists and other professionals need to have a clear understanding of the various pathologies. Gynecological causes include less and more common as well as acute and chronic pathologies, as summarized in Table 3. Different lower back pathologies (vertebral nerve, discopathy) can also often lead to pelvic pain, emphasizing that these diagnoses should take into account low back and the symptoms of both. Understanding this points can help selecting investigations and treatments, thus accelerating the diagnostic process.

The following are gynecological causes for pelvic and lower back pain, which are particularly important to consider. An ectopic pregnancy can cause pain in the lower back, hips, and thighs on one side of the body, and more generalized abdominal pain. Fibroids can cause pelvic pain or lower back pain in different ways, such as via menstrual pain. Dysmenorrhea is pain during menstruation, which might appear in the abdomen, pelvis, lower back, and/or upper thighs. Ovulation pain is caused by the reduction of the follicle, which can stretch the surface of the ovary, causing pain in that region—namely, in the lower abdomen and occasionally in the lower back as well. Amenorrhea (absence of menstruation) is a concerning symptom for many women. It can be related to weight changes, irregular birth control use, hormonal imbalances, polycystic ovary syndrome, and perimenopause (approaching menopause). Pelvic inflammatory disease (PID) is frequently associated with endometriosis. These adhesions manifest in the form of sharp, nagging pain, which can increase with movement—resulting in muscle pain in the lower back or upper region. Ovarian cyst pain is associated with a lower backache, accentuated during menstrual periods and sexual intercourse, and presents with irregular periods. UTI, STD, and other infections can cause pelvic pain and can also cause stabbing pain in the lower back. Vaginal yeast infection symptoms can include painful urination or sex, generalized itching, and pain during intercourse, consequently causing lower back pain. Endometriosis can present with deep pelvic and lower pain. Pelvic inflammatory disease can sometimes present with lower back pain alongside generalized pelvic pain.

3.3. Urological Causes

Urinary patients report discomfort and increased symptoms while sitting for a long time, especially while driving. Some patients have pain from a feeling of fluid in it, pain when touched, and voiding, so they treat physical therapy as normal. On average, when treating physical therapy, filling the fluid in the seminal vesicles is very rare. Even if you have a symptom report, it is impossible to confirm whether the problem is occurring from the urinary system and to validate the treatment effect (since the symptoms can increase and the filling test cannot be performed).

When a patient is found to have urinary symptoms, they are advised to investigate urinary and urological causes first. Symptoms include dysuria, increased abdominal pain during micturition or defecation, urinary frequency, urinary incontinence, urinary hesitancy, and straining to begin urination, mild suprapubic or perineal pain immediately after voiding, and urinary pain, cloudiness, or the presence of mucus close to the urine.

Some patients report pain between their penises and anuses, which is connected to the pelvic area. The feeling of "I feel like I'm going to pee myself" can exacerbate the patient's anxiety and pain. Some may experience pain in the lower back.

3.4. Digestive Causes

Hind or front or side abdominal lining, in fact. There are some important minus signs to suggest that this effect could be directly exerted upon the back brakes and the tissues secured to the brake piston (meaning any or all of...). Also, the pelvis feathers could plausibly be disturbed in this manner, though for a wider variety of ways than the brake system. Nausea of the severity and type associated with gastritis can be associated with increased activity of the diaphragm serratus muscle and muscles of shoulder blade fixation, as well as the upper neck muscles. The neural network that likely drives this feedback is called the "emotive mode" flow stack, and it is really excellently handy in our experience at devising permanent and painful postural accommodations to a range of mostly slow, lazy, and latent problems. Given the more direct and closely anatomical relationships between the mid-bottom and these removal flows, this feedback is more about indicating the likely extent of the problem than anything else. Feedback based purely on nervous system activity tends to be fairly "gut" oriented, though progression of disease can lead to physical stress on surrounding tissues. Now bear in mind that the area of greatest mechanoreceptive feedback in the back, pelvis, and front abdominal wall relative to the digestive system is very specific. And then, in unusual, chronic cancers of the several digestive glands...

The specific subset of the digestive system that we think we are talking about when we talk about digesting is actually only one of two that has direct physical contact with colloids passing through the gut tube. The key players here are the secretions of the exocrine portion of those glands, each of which has direct contact with the small intestine during a real "digestion as chemical processing" function. Perhaps most notably, as opposed to the direct physical processing done at every part of detergic action, the chemical processing properties are unique in the gastrointestinal system. The chemical properties of the termini small intestine make the neural and muscular functions that control this section uniquely responsive to the chemical factors that enter into this mix. For this reason, the cells of the mucosal lining of the gastrointestinal system that release these chemicals in our experience are targeted as often as anything else in the rest of the gut tube for chemotherapy. Theoretically, the pelvic floor, wall, or back could see a wide variety of slow and latent problems from the toxicity syndrome that could affect any of that.

Because the digestive system is a high volume source of a wide variety of biochemicals and can cause an especially wide and troublesome variety of symptoms, digestive causes of pelvic pain are theoretically more likely to be correlated with pelvic floor pain, back pain, and others. Understand that the physiology of each digestive organ is unique and will undoubtedly vary in no small degree from individual to individual, but the thematic similarities become disproportionately obvious when you begin to look at them in the (more or less holistic) mental model promoted within this document.

4. Diagnosis and Assessment of Pelvic and Lower Back Pain

There are no blood tests or imaging studies that can prove that pain is coming from a specific back problem. However, your healthcare provider may choose to order tests to determine the cause of the back or pelvic pain or to help set a plan for pain management. A physical examination might be made of you, including an examination of your back and your pelvis. Such a test is conducted by a medical professional, usually a doctor, who is testing different muscles, body functioning, and pain, touching the lower back and starting the movements. The evaluation also checks the lower parts of the back, as well as the muscles, tissues, nerves, cartilage, and bones that collaborate in the area's workings. Doctors can look for three main different things with such tests, using them to help draw conclusions and make a diagnosis.

Once you explain your symptoms to a healthcare provider, they will perform a thorough assessment and examination that focuses on the back and pelvis. It is important that healthcare providers use your narrative as the basis for their examinations and not solely rely on the physical exam findings. Imaging studies, such as X-rays and MRI, are often ordered for patients with severe, unremitting pain such as that of sciatica or in cases where nerve compression is suspected. Laboratory testing, including a complete blood cell count, electrolytes, tests for diabetes, systemic lupus erythematosus, ankylosing spondylitis, and proteinuria, among others, is done if warranted by symptoms or the medical history.

4.1. Physical Examination

In the clinic, the evaluation of pelvic pain and lower back pain is primarily focused on identifying the source of pain. If the source of the pain disappears, the pain reproduction factor can be used to decide the test and treatment options. Therefore, a thorough physical examination of the pelvis and lower back should be conducted to determine the various pain generators. Pelvic floor muscles in the assessment of pelvic girdle pain are not always considered; however, they can be a potential source of musculoskeletal and myofascial pain. Muscles involved in the pelvic girdle are most responsible for pain, while bony landmarks and sacroiliac joint pain are less responsible due to the nerve supply that connects the pelvic floor muscles. This review discusses an up-to-date comprehensive examination of pelvic and/or lower back pain in various existing studies.

Physical examination of patients presenting with pelvic and/or lower back pain is an essential part of the evaluation. In a standard medical or physical therapy visit, patients visit healthcare professionals in search of a diagnosis and effective treatments. In some cases, exam findings can direct healthcare professionals toward the most effective course of action for the patients. In the examination process, objective measures are assessed using physical maneuvers and observations. These methods can potentially assist in locating the pain origin and appropriate treatments. Collectively, the authors discuss a comprehensive examination and review specific assessment tools of the pelvis that can be beneficial in assessing and treating patients with pelvic pain and/or lower back pain. An assessment team method can be used in examinations; however, patient factors such as comfort levels and confounding factors can affect whether or not there is a complete assessment.

4.2. Imaging Studies

The first technique used is X-ray. X-rays of the pelvis and of the lumbo-sacral, coated in the bending theoretical either standard flexible frontal lateral. A second level exam can be suggested by the orthopedic surgeon and/or radiologist. It is the MRI, useful to show better almost all neighboring noble structures. This examination must be returned to if the patient still very young (to exclude dysplasia coxo femoral) presented with clinical aspects that may be consistent with neoplastic, infectious, degenerative, enthesic, hormonal, traumatic, vegetarian diseases. It is necessary to exclude both common and rare causes of mechanical coxalgia or acute or chronic sacro-iliac pain. It is necessary to combine basic radiographic and magnetic imaging investigations with a good clinical acumen and the palpation of painful reactivations and periarticular inflamed tissue on the osteoarticular level.

Imaging studies are useful to support the diagnosis, especially when the existence of a lesion or a musculoskeletal disease is suspected, and in cases of apparent refractory myofascial pain, in some cases of spinal stenosis, disc degeneration, or herniation. MRI and electrodiagnostic studies such as EMG can help identify the specific source of the structural or anatomical changes, which are not usually the sole factor or explanation of pain. The images may be better to warn us of the diseases that can coexist and contribute to mechanical environments such as inflammatory, ischemic, nutritional, autoimmune injuries. In general, imaging techniques are well suited for the diagnosis of neoplastic, infectious, rheumatological, endocrine, vascular, traumatic, and/or degenerative diseases. Imaging techniques are also used in studies to show tissues and organs to identify morphological, structural, functional, or pathological states.

4.3. Laboratory Tests

Diagnosis includes presence of characteristic symptoms, signs in clinical examination and imaging. Laboratory test is not necessary in the majority of cases but in some situations it is helpful. Laboratory test includes general tests such as white blood cell (WBC) in the blood, C-reactive protein (CRP) in the blood, erythrocyte sedimentation rate (ESR) in the blood. Estimation of some special biochemical and physiological marker are locally obtained from the urine (soluble transferrin receptor, immunoreactive hepcidin and uromodulin) are beneficial in the evaluation of this diseases. On the other hand, from synovial fluid, radiological images and serum venous useful markers are the protein carbonyl levels, interleukin 6 and metalloproteinase among tissue inhibitors of metalloproteinase, and immunoreactive hepcidin. In addition, neurobiological components are estimated and are not as specific as currently supposed. A liver estimation, such as the enzymes Toll-like receptors and myeloperoxidase, should be practiced on or tend to injure persons to exclude attempts to conceal the use of different drugs.

As with imaging studies, laboratory tests are also indicated in only selected cases. In conclusion, in patients presenting with symptoms of pelvic pain and/or lower back pain, a detailed patient history and clinical examination should be carefully conducted to clearly diagnose, enable differential diagnosis, or identify potentially dangerous conditions that may simulate symptoms of pelvic pain and lower back pain. No laboratory tests provide a 100% degree of certainty in the diagnosis of painful endometriosis and strongly corroborate the findings of clinical history and gynecological examination. Despite the existence of normal "biochemical and physiological markers" from patients with pain, the majority of them present changes such as the modifications of the immune system on multiple in and organ system.

5. Conventional Treatment Options

These include: acetaminophen, NSAIDs (ibuprofen, naproxen), oral muscle relaxants, some antidepressants, and others. NSAIDs are the recommended first choice for pain relief, rather than paracetamol (acetaminophen) (e.g., ibuprofen and naproxen) or muscle relaxers. Medications may provide some relief when taken as part of a comprehensive treatment plan but are not regarded as a standalone cure for back or pelvic pain by themselves. Injections: Some chronic lower back pain patients may benefit from prescribing corticosteroid injections, nerve blocks, or other medications to reduce inflammation and reduce pain. After a thorough examination and discussion with their healthcare provider, patients may be directed toward several injection methods that effectively deliver anti-inflammatory drugs to nerve roots that may be causing discomfort. Surgery: In rare situations, extreme pain or loss of function due to injury or wear and tear can necessitate an operation. If surgery is considered, several discussions with a healthcare provider are recommended, as well as medical assessments to ensure the procedure is safe.

Pelvic and lower back pain must be accurately diagnosed in order to identify the primary source of the problem and provide the most effective treatment. A tailor-made recovery plan that takes into account an individual's pain, activity level, and overall health is a good first step towards chronic pain patients finding some relief. Available therapies can be divided into non-pharmacological therapies, medications, injections, and surgery. Non-drug treatments and self-care techniques, such as heat or ice, yoga, tai chi, or physical therapy centered on stretching, walking, or swimming, are included in the non-pharmacological choices. These treatments need to be performed in conjunction with other treatments to be effective.

5.1. Medications

Model guidance for the CNS-CRN developed by NICE Interventional Procedures Program (2020) is summarized in Table 7. Several medications are used with limited evidence of efficacy for the treatment of pelvic girdle pain and are therefore not shown.

In some circumstances, when the pain is localized or also affecting the upper back, neuropathic pain therapies such as amitriptyline, pregabalin, and gabapentin can be used.

Spinal opiates such as morphine may be offered to patients with lower back pain when first- and second-line treatments have been exhausted and all the following criteria are satisfied: a) Persistent pain of severe intensity. b) Neuropathic and nociceptive pain in suffering patients. c) The impact of the pain is significant, with adverse consequences.

Opiates are also suggested for neuropathic pain in herpes zoster affecting the lower back, which is a mixture of neuropathic and nociceptive pain. Tramadol, which influences the normal and altered transmission and modulation of pain mainly through opioid receptors and other systems in the central nervous system, can be used.

Tramadol is a synthetic opioid mainly derived from the metabolization of the parent medications codeine and N-desmethyltramadol. Opioid analgesics are used in adult patients to manage chronic pain and neuropathic pain associated with neurological conditions.

Neuropathic pain is predominantly controlled with membrane-stabilizing medications such as certain antidepressants (duloxetine, venlafaxine) and tricyclic antidepressants (e.g., nortriptyline, amitriptyline), as well as certain anticonvulsants like pregabalin and gabapentin.

Pelvic pain, similar to chronic lower back pain, is pharmacologically managed by a multidisciplinary team. The treatment consists mostly of antipyretics, analgesics, and anti-inflammatory drugs. Analgesics are medications that effectively address pain by targeting both nociceptive and neuropathic pathways.

5.1 Medications

5.2. Physical Therapy

Active Treatment Options Multiple manual therapy methods to treat SIJD can be used. Traction (pulling the bones of the body away from each other) can help "gap" the joint to create space in the joint and decrease pain. Muscle energy is a manual therapy technique commonly used in the lumbar spine to restore proper joint mechanics and decrease pain. When the sacral bones are stuck, a common area that becomes painful is the pubic symphysis joint in the front of the pelvis. In individuals with pubic symphysis pain, manipulation to the bones of the pelvis may help improve range of motion and decrease pain over time. In addition to manual techniques, there are several exercises and movements included as part of the treatment for pelvic pain. These exercises are used to simultaneously stabilize and mobilize the pelvis. The clamshell exercise can help to stabilize the pelvis and increase hip strength, which decompresses the low back and can decrease pain.

It is important to remember that for people with pelvic pain symptoms or chronic lower back pain, often one dysfunctional area worsens pain in the other area. Physical therapy frequently integrates treatment of both the lumbar spine and/or pelvis simultaneously to decrease pain. This will present as a holistic or whole-body approach to pain management that is individual to each patient. Treatment often includes manual therapies, mobilizations, manipulations, myofascial release techniques, and various exercises, including general stabilization and strengthening exercises targeting the core, glutes, and hips. The overall goal is to improve and complement another area's function to alleviate or improve in chronic pelvic and lower back pain.

5.3. Injections

An injection containing anesthetic agents or saline with steroid may be administered into the sore and swollen joint. This helps confirm that the symptoms arise from the joint. The steroids may help reduce the pain and inflammation.

5.3.2. Facet joint injections

Caudal: The injection occurs through the sacral opening of the spine, directing medication to the nerve roots traveling through the spinal canal adjacent to the bone where the nerves get squeezed. This approach is less common but used in certain cases. People with low back pain, as well as leg pain, may benefit from this approach.

Transforaminal: The needle is placed via the side of the vertebral bodies, targeting the epidural space and draining the nerve roots. This approach allows the solution to stay local to the nerves, increasing efficacy. This approach is preferred by most practitioners for treating sciatica.

Interlaminar: The injection occurs in the back central portion of the vertebrae called the laminae, just outside the dura, around the irritated spinal nerves. This approach is common for low back or neck pain patients.

Preparations of medications (corticosteroids) or a mix of medications and a therapeutic relief substance (anesthetic agents) are injected inside the spine, targeting the area around the spinal cord or nerves. The goal is to help reduce swelling of the affected spinal nerves, leading to a downstream reduction in pain symptoms and enabling physical therapy compliance. There are several different approaches for the administration of epidural steroid injections, which include:

5.3.1. Epidural steroid injections

6. Complementary and Alternative Therapies

Chiropractic care has been reported to be beneficial to patients with pelvic girdle pain complaints. Three primary clinical changes took place over the 16 weeks of therapy: pain decreased and function improved. A statistically significant improvement was shown in the amount of pain, twist endurance, and self-reported disability, with 40% of patients showing a 50% reduction in pain at week 4 of treatment, and 95% experiencing an 85% reduction at week 16. Based on the present results and limited previous research, chiropractic adjustments in the pelvic and lumbosacral region are supported as an acceptable non-drug, non-invasive, and non-surgical approach. Massage therapy improves symptoms of lumbopelvic pain during pregnancy. A study established the aim that evaluation of the effectiveness that massage therapy plays in the reduction of lumbopelvic pain in pregnancy in comparison to its medical therapy. It was found that the study conducted showed that massage therapy reduces lumbopelvic pain and symptoms of Pregnancy-related Lumbopelvic Pain, such as depressive symptoms, problems with movement, and sleep, and general quality and life, in a more significant way, compared to physical medicine alone. Thus, it provides sufficient evidence that massage therapy is effective in treatment options for morphia Pelvic and LBP during pregnancy.

Acupuncture can be applied in the treatment of pelvic pain. Needles inserted into the skin at different areas in the body can modify the way the spinal cord transmits the sensation of pain. In a recent review, conducted in 2017, two researchers analyzed the clinical trial studies of laser acupuncture which operates with light emitting diode needle system and which stimulate near acupuncture lasers. These lasers do not make a point and are more simple. The result shows that this kind of treatment relieves Pelvic Girdle Pain during pregnancy and reported an improvement in lumbar position and increase the bed activities, but more studies are required in this new field.

6.1. Acupuncture

A licensed expert sometimes administers a safer form of acupuncture known as electro-acupuncture. In addition to supporting traditional practice, electro-acupuncture is thought to alter the ways in which pain is interpreted by the brain. Acupuncture has been thought to offer discomfort relief in people with some other kinds of arthritis, as it reduces muscle spasms and calms the body. However, there is no scientific evidence to support this claim. More study is required to establish the function of acupuncture in the care of people with pelvic and back ache. Although the National Institute of Good Practice in the U.K. suggests that results may be signs of a mental illness, several advanced treatment restoration strategies already involve acupuncture. Some patients have reported decreased pain after using acupuncture.

While acupuncture is an ancient traditional Chinese medicine (TCM) practice, it wasn't a very familiar concept in the West until very recently. The practice of acupuncture uses the insertion of very thin needles through the patient's skin, at specific points throughout the body. As a natural, safe, and effective method of treatment, acupuncture has been used for over five thousand years. For some patients with pelvic and back pain, acupuncture may be a safe and beneficial option. Many people seek out this complementary therapy for persistent chronic back pain. While scientific evidence is unclear whether acupuncture is effective in controlling chronic pain, acupuncture may deliver positive results when combined with other pelvic pain management options.

6.2. Chiropractic Care

Chiropractors are licensed healthcare providers who take an evidence-informed, patient-centered approach to care for pelvic and/or low back pain (and other related complaints). The intent of chiropractic treatment is to correct imbalances or poor movement in the spinal column and/or other anatomical structures (fascia, ligaments, tendons, muscles) of the body, which may interfere with the function of the nervous system, posture, movement, balance, and activities of daily living. Chiropractors have a variety of treatment options available, known as the "menu of services." One of the most common and widely recognized procedures provided by chiropractors is manual adjustment or manipulation of the low back or pelvis. There are many types of spinal adjustments or manipulation techniques employed by chiropractors, and training and proficiency may vary. In general, a chiropractic adjustment is delivered by hand and involves a quick thrust to a restricted joint with the intended goal of increasing range of motion, improving function, and pain reduction. The effects of a chiropractic adjustment may be local, at the treatment site, or systemic, affecting a patient's well-being and overall quality of life. The evidence suggests short-term relief of pelvic and/or lower back pain with the use of chiropractic spinal manipulation as a treatment option.

Chiropractic care has been described as the third most utilized complementary and alternative medicine in the United States. Chiropractic care focuses on the diagnosis and management of musculoskeletal conditions with a focus on conservative management. Chiropractors commonly perform a series of manual, non-pharmacological interventions when treating patients in a chiropractic clinic. Chiropractic care could be beneficial in patients who suffer pelvic and/or low back pain and wish to visit a provider with particular training and expertise related to the musculoskeletal system who can deliver these non-pharmacological interventions.

6.3. Massage Therapy

There are a number of theories on how massage therapy may work. It has been suggested that the application to the soft tissues may work to reduce pain by sending signals to the brain that compete with the signal of pain. Massage therapy is also considered to help relax muscles and improve blood flow to an area of problem by using mild pressure and known to enhance the removal of toxins from muscle tissue. Massage therapy can also have a psychological effect, increasing a person's feeling of relaxation and reducing tension.

We are not aware of any UK guidelines for chronic or acute pelvic or low back pain that recommend massage therapy. However, the guidelines reviewed for our systematic review had a section on manual therapies, including massage therapy. Massage therapists may work within a variety of settings and can specialize in various types of massage therapy. Various authors have noted that massage therapists use different techniques. These may include: effleurage (using the hands to apply stroking movements to the back), petrissage (kneading movements similar to those used in baking bread), friction (pressing across the fibers), percussion/vibration (rhythmic tapping or vibration movements) and minor joint movements.

Massage therapy is a complementary therapy that is used in a variety of healthcare settings. Massage therapy involves the use of manual techniques, such as applying fixed or movable pressure, rubbing, rolling, rocking, and holding of tissues within the area of pain, to manipulate the soft tissues of the body. These techniques can be performed with or without the use of oils, lotions, powders, or other preparations. The purpose of these manipulative techniques is to reduce the pain experienced. Massage techniques can also be used in combination with other complementary therapy approaches.

7. Lifestyle Modifications for Managing Pelvic and Lower Back Pain

Research suggests that a diet high in processed foods, sugar, caffeine, alcohol, and smoking contribute to pelvic/low back pain. Some believe when inflamed and acidic, the nerve fibers are more likely to perceive low back and pelvic pain. Maintaining an anti-inflammatory diet will help to reduce or eliminate pelvic and low back pain. Diagnosing at our office with a pH test strip and nudging the patient in the direction of eliminating the sugar and unnatural chemicals from their diet has consistently shown positive responses. Providing the patient with a good meal plan at the beginning of their care indicating the importance of reducing inflammation/alkalizing the body is an important step to help them recover from this pain.

Diet and Nutrition

Those who have chronic pelvic pain have a tendency to also develop pelvic girdle muscle weakness. Specific stretching, strengthening, and stabilizing of the pelvis is an important tool in reducing pelvic and low back pain. In the beginning stages of rehabilitation, the patient may begin a basic isometric therapy for the UR pelvic stabilizers. A physical therapist will have to instruct/demonstrate proper technique and execution to avoid other muscle groups compensating.

Exercise, Stretch, and Exercise More

Good ergonomics and posture are an integral part of managing any kind of pain. Whether it's from repetitive movements, lifting, or daily life, poor posture and ergonomics will always make any kind of pain worse. Once you have taken time off work for a few weeks or months, it is important that when you return to work, that ergonomics and posture are addressed so that you don't cause further injury or inflammation.

Ergonomics and Posture

7.1. Ergonomics and Posture

Lifestyle: Ergonomics and Posture. Ergonomics and Posture are modifications that improve task efficiency and increase a person's ability to put spaces and things to good use. This concept is created to help the environment fit the people to decrease the negative impact of the task. This concept has been mostly applied to the job environment, but it is possible to use this concept to adapt many environments over a 24-hour period. "Bad" body mechanics and postures are not inherently bad. Every body has its own comfortable way to reside and move. What is important is that excessive strain and work can cause musculoskeletal weaknesses and chronic pain. Changing the way to attain a habit or posture that promotes a better-supported body can also reduce or prevent chronic pain.

Making changes to your lifestyle can help control and prevent a lot of pelvic, abdominal, and lower back pain. First, you need to look at your living and work environments for toxic exposures, hormone disruptors, acid-forming foods, and ergonomics/posture issues. Just about everything in our life – from the way you hold your grocery bags to the way you sit at your computer – can slowly erode your body and create chronic pain. These lifestyle changes have a significant impact on endometriosis and adenomyosis. Anything that can minimize the pain and inflammation can lengthen the time between surgeries and can even help prevent the need for surgery.

7.2. Exercise and Stretching

Incorporating stretching into a daily routine can be highly effective in managing pelvic and lower back pain. Strive for a minimum of 30 minutes of effective stretching and exercise routines for at least four to five days a week. Progressive stretching (with appropriate warm-ups and cool downs) will increase overall flexibility and strength. Studies also indicate that a gentle warm yoga class once a week can improve long-term flexibility, stretching, attunement to the body and mind connection, and relaxation. Tensing the muscles in a stretching routine for a count of 20-30 seconds at three to five-second intervals is an effective strategy. discuss a comprehensive stretching and deep tissue myofascial release routine for the conservative improvement of pelvic and lower-back pain. Furthermore, they provide recommendations for arcuate stretching, a deep tissue myofascial program, stretching, and core exercises to stabilize the lumbar spine.

Stretching

Low-intensity and low-impact physical activity, such as walking, swimming, and biking, can help increase stamina and overall well-being. It is important to tailor physical activity to a comfort level that promotes endurance and overall improvement. It is important to start slow and listen to the body's pain signals to optimize strengthening and rehabilitation. Identify activities that are attainable and can be advanced incrementally week after week. Studies show that a sedentary or inactive lifestyle can lead to enteric nervous system hypersensitivity and thus increase lower-back pain. Tailoring an exercise program to target the enteric and somatic nervous systems can promote a decrease in centralized pain, hypertonicity, spasm, weakness, and deconditioning.

Exercise

7.3. Diet and Nutrition

A lower DII was associated with a 2-year reduced risk of developing low back pain in one study conducted with middle-aged adults. In a population-based study conducted in Australia, the highest risk of low back pain was associated with low intake of dietary antioxidants. Individuals with osteoarthritis of the knee and low back pain have also been found to have low vitamin D receptor expression. There have been no intervention studies with pelvic low back pain patients evaluating the effects of omega-3 fatty acids, which appear to play a role in minimizing systemic inflammation. These studies appear to have focused on diet as a lifestyle modification. A study by Christian et al. involved a multi-modal intervention including diets, whereas the other studies included a high-fat diet that is more appropriate for cancer patients who may have unintended weight loss. More studies focusing on diet, which target individuals who are not obese, are needed to increase our understanding of the role of modifiable dietary factors that might impact musculoskeletal pain states.

Cross-sectional studies of community-based samples with operative management of the pain state suggest that individuals who are obese tend to have increased odds of low back pain and spine osteoarthritis. Additionally, weight loss has been associated with a reduction in pain in research trials. Though current cumulative data suggests that weight loss can be helpful in decreasing pelvic and low back pain, modifiable dietary factors may also play a role in decreasing musculoskeletal pain. Dietary inflammatory index (DII) is a measure of the inflammatory potential of an individual's diet. Currently, there are two articles discussing the positive association between elevated levels of systemic inflammation and back pain in those individuals with the highest inflammatory index.

8. Psychological Strategies for Coping with Chronic Pain

- From this neuropsychobiological perspective, numerous psychological interventions have been developed that target the emotional and motivational dimensions of chronic pain. CBT, ACT, DBT, Metacognitive Therapy are examples of a range of approaches that seek to help individuals connect to their emotions with courage and compassion. Systematic reviews of outcome research suggest that psychological treatment that focuses on self-acceptance and values-based living alongside strategies to manage and regulate emotions are more effective than interventions that seek to reduce emotional experience or avoid emotions. Helping people develop emotional regulation skills has been found to be highly beneficial as part of a broader treatment model regardless of the intensity and impact of the emotions themselves. For example, developing compassion for oneself and others can help improve pain, disability, and depression in the context of chronic pain.

Emotional dimensions of pain and strategies to manage emotions - Addressing emotional distress has been a neglected component of pain care for many years. In the past, psychological treatment focused on reducing negative emotions, which entailed the challenging position of trivializing the individual's lived experience of pain and their emotional responses to it. Finally, anger or aggression were directed inwards, towards the self, with emotions such as fear, anxiety, and sadness perceived as being an out-of-control response to pain that needed to be modified alongside the actual levels of pain. In contrast to this perspective, today we understand that pain and the emotional core of our being are inseparable.

9. Preventive Measures and Strategies to Avoid Recurrence

Given that sugar can play a role in the development of inflammation, reducing sugar intake may also be advantageous. It may be beneficial to decrease the amount of processed and refined meals in your diet and to eat fewer fast food items. As previously stated, it is advisable to seek the guidance of a dietician to develop and plan a diet that is appropriate for you and your needs. Drinking enough water every day is important in keeping ligaments, discs, and joints nourished and in sound health. At the very least, eight 8oz glasses of water should be consumed every day, but if possible, more. All of the suggestions mentioned here can be beneficial in not only preventing pelvic or lower back pain from occurring, but also in helping one to live a healthier lifestyle, which will keep you feeling and functioning well. It has been demonstrated that healthcare plans that incorporate physical activity intervention techniques have a beneficial effect on the life and work of injured patients. Such efforts have been shown to result in a greater restoration of typical actions, a greater capacity to cope with day-to-day tasks, and a greater capacity to cope with work. As a result, strive to incorporate this knowledge into everyday work with patients suffering from stiff or aching pelvic girdles or lower backs.

To reduce the risk of experiencing lower back or pelvic pain, a plethora of proactive approaches can be adopted. Strengthening the lower back, abdominal, pelvic, and hip muscles, as well as the muscles that provide spinal support, is an excellent approach. However, hip and pelvic flexibility must not be overlooked. Aside from obtaining regular cardiovascular exercise to improve circulation, it is equally critical to remember that regular physical activity and mobility help to keep the body pliable. Make efforts to get up and stretch if you sit for lengthy periods. Find a standing workstation if possible, as sitting for prolonged periods can exacerbate your condition. Inflammation can make your symptoms worse, so it's important to avoid or manage it if it occurs. While the advantages of anti-inflammatory agents have previously been discussed, decreasing the number of inflammatory agents consumed through the diet might also be beneficial. There are several types of berries and seeds that are high in antioxidants and low in pro-inflammatory elements. When selecting cooking oils, opt for those low in omega-6 fatty acids but high in omega-3. Maintain a balanced diet with a variety of plant-based foods to nourish your body.

10. Emerging Technologies and Innovations in Pelvic and Lower Back Pain Management

Emerging technologies in pelvic and lower back pain management have a long future. The likely future innovations include a complete replacement of currently popular state-of-the-art therapies such as expanded intelligent pain pump, neuronavigation diagnosis systems for endoscopic ultrasound-guided suprachoroidal block and TAP blocks, and neoteric genetic pain diagnostics. Although we have noted a burgeoning flow of patients who have high pain hypersensitivities who are responding fabulously to pharmacologic therapies of Sumatriptan with TXA. More studies in cost vs risk need to be assessed in this area with larger clinical trials which could also involve evaluation of minimally invasive neuromodulation technology. Also, despite enormous years of cumulative experience, we are still learning more on pelvic nerve system variations and pathoanatomy taking the aid of advanced MRIs and genetics. A huge potential remains with artificial intelligence for image interpretation and heat mapping such as parasonic and pixelsensor. Last, but not least, protocols still have been improved in continued validation for multidisciplinary treatment regimes with technologies such as pain pebble.

Recent years have witnessed several advancements in the field of pelvic and lower back pain management. These innovations in the management of chronic pelvic and lower back pain hold great promise and have the potential to change treatment paradigms for these challenging conditions. The field of pain management is witnessing a rapid, steep rise in innovative improvements, but these areas have not been covered in most of the existing prime medical literature on postoperative pelvic and lower back pain managing strategies. As a matter of fact, most of these are reports or case series, and their use is endorsed by consensus and expert opinion. The therapeutic interventions and emerging technologies for the treatment of pelvic and lower back pain have several applications, and many of these techniques have shown positive outcomes in the management of acute as well as chronic pelvic and lower back pain. Recent endoscopic ultrasound-guided or pararectus TAP block, erector spinae plane block, quadratus lumborum block, and platelet-rich plasma therapies are emerging as innovations in postoperative pelvic and lower back pain relief.

11. Patient Education and Empowerment

We also previously reported a robust relationship between greater patient education regarding options available to them and behavioral engagement in all modes of self-management. Because the Pain Rehabilitation Center (PRC) approach to steading pain encompasses multiple therapeutic models for the individual, meaningful education in an identified learning style may serve to improve access to additional services for patients. Besides the importance of optimized patient outcomes, our interest and involvement in patient education at the PRC lies in its ability to create a continuum of access to, and interest in, peer support programming, options and functions. We want our patients to take their health into their own hands, supported when needed. Our aim is to cultivate participants with the confidence to start and maintain an individualized self-management journey of their choice for years to come.

Many experts in pain rehabilitation believe that patient education is one of the most crucial areas of clinical practice. We want our patients to be empowered future consumers of treatments—only undergoing procedures and interventions when they are fully informed and feel that they are making an important and informed choice. This type of shared decision-making underscores the collaboration that we believe is important between patients and providers. Our job as clinicians is not only to do the procedures and execute medication management, but to educate about pain and help individuals learn to self-manage. Patient education can also serve as a therapeutic medium, providing a level of prevention for additional mental health disorders - for example in the instance of avoiding extended periods of social withdrawal or periods of feeling increasingly isolated.

www.ingramcontent.com/pod-product-compliance
Lightning Source LLC
Chambersburg PA
CBHW070810260726
48660CB00005B/1795